The Ultimate Pegan Diet Cookbook for Beginners

Lose Weight and Burn Fat Faster with The Fastest Pegan Diet Recipe Collection

Emy Fit

Table of Contents

Classic Apple Oats 6

Peach & Chia Seed 8

Avocado Spread..10

Almond Butter and Blueberry Smoothie 12

Salmon and Egg Muffins..14

Stuffed Celery..16

Butternut Squash Fries 18

Dried Fig Tapenade 20

Speedy Sweet Potato Chips 22

Nachos with Hummus (Mediterranean Inspired) 23

Hummus and Olive Pita Bread 25

Roast Asparagus 26

Chicken Kale Wraps..28

Tomato Triangles..30

Zaatar Fries..32

Summertime Vegetable Chicken Wraps..34

Premium Roasted Baby Potatoes..36

Tomato and Cherry Linguine 38

Mediterranean Zucchini Mushroom Pasta.....................................40

Lemon and Garlic Fettucine 42

Roasted Broccoli with Parmesan..44

Spinach and Feta Bread 46

Quick Zucchini Bowl 48

Healthy Basil Platter..50

Tomato Bruschetta...51

Artichoke Flatbread 53

Red Pepper Tapenade 55

Coriander Falafel 57

Cinnamon and Hemp Seed Coffee Shake......................................60

Green Smoothie 62

Strawberry and Banana Smoothie... 64

Orange Smoothie 66

Pumpkin Chai Smoothie 68

Banana Shake... 70

Green Honeydew Smoothie 72

Summer Salsa... 74

Red Salsa.. 76

Pinto Bean Dip... 78

Smoky Red Pepper Hummus 80

Spinach Dip.. 82

Tomatillo Salsa 84

Arugula Pesto Couscous 86

Oatmeal and Raisin Balls... 88

Nacho Cheese... 90

Pico de Gallo.. 92

Moroccan-Style Couscous with Chickpeas................................. 94

Vegetarian Paella with Green Beans and Chickpeas 96

Garlic Prawns with Tomatoes and Basil...................................... 98

Stuffed Calamari in Tomato Sauce 100

Provencal Braised Hake.. 102

Pan-Roasted Sea Bass.. 104

Delicious Quinoa & Dried 106

Classic Apple Oats

Preparation Time: 10 minutes

Cooking Time: 15 minutes

Servings: 2

Ingredients:

- ½ tsp. cinnamon
- ¼ tsp. ginger
- 2 apples make half-inch chunks
- ½ c. oats, steel cut
- 1½ c. water
- Maple syrup
- ¼ tsp. salt
- Clove
- ¼ tsp. nutmeg

Directions:

1. Take Instant Pot and careful y arrange it over a clean, dry kitchen platform.
2. Turn on the appliance.
3. In the cooking pot area, add the water, oats, cinnamon, ginger, clove, nutmeg, apple, and salt. Stir the ingredients gently.

4. Close the pot lid and seal the valve to avoid any leakage. Find and press the "Manual" cooking setting and set cooking time to 5 minutes.
5. Allow the recipe ingredients to cook for the set time, and after that, the timer reads "zero."
6. Press "Cancel" and press "NPR" setting for natural pressure release. It takes 8-10 times for all inside pressure to release.
7. Open the pot and arrange the cooked recipe in serving plates.
8. Sweeten as needed with maple or agave syrup and serve immediately.
9. Top with some chopped nuts, optional.

Nutrition:

Calories: 232,

Fat: 5.7 g,

Carbs: 48.1 g,

Protein: 5.2 g 66

Peach & Chia Seed

Preparation Time: 10 minutes

Cooking Time: 10 minutes

Servings: 2

Ingredients:

- ½ oz. chia seeds

- 1 tbsp. pure maple syrup

- 1 c. coconut milk

- 1 tsp. ground cinnamon

- 3 diced peaches

- 2/3 c. granola

Directions:

1. Find a small bowl and add the chia seeds, maple syrup, and coconut milk.

2. Stir well, then cover and pop into the fridge for at least one hour.

3. Find another bowl, add the peaches and sprinkle with the cinnamon. Pop to one side

4. When it's time to serve, take two glasses, and pour the chia mixture between the two.

5. Sprinkle the granola over the top, keeping a tiny amount to one side to use to decorate later.

6. Top with the peaches and top with the reserved granola and serve.

Nutrition:

Calories: 415,

Protein: 13.9g,

Carbs: 54.4g,

Fat: 16.9g 68

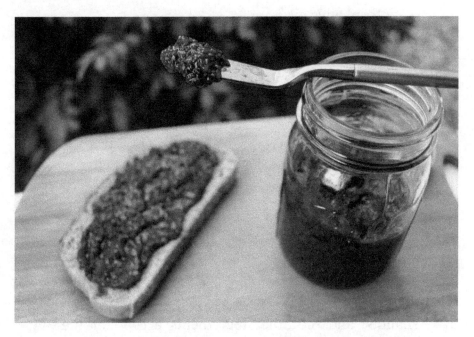

Avocado Spread

Preparation Time: 10 minutes

Cooking Time: 1 minutes

Servings: 2

Ingredients:

- 2 peeled and pitted avocados

- 1 tbsp. olive oil

- 1 tbsp. minced shallots

- 1 tbsp. lime juice

- 1 tbsp. heavy coconut cream

- Salt

- Black pepper

- 1 tbsp. chopped chives

Directions:
1. In a blender, combine the avocado flesh with the oil, shallots, and the other ingredients except for the chopped chives.

2. Pulse well, divide into bowls, sprinkle the chives on top, and serve as a morning spread.

Nutrition:

Calories: 79,

Fat: 0.4 g,

Carbs: 15 g,

Protein: 1.3 g 71

Almond Butter and Blueberry Smoothie

Preparation Time: 10 minutes

Cooking Time: 1 minutes

Servings: 2

Ingredients:

- 1 c. almond milk

- 1 c. blueberries

- 4 ice cubes

- 1 scoop vanilla protein powder

- 1 tbsp. almond butter

- 1 tbsp. chia seeds

Directions:

1. Use a blender to mix the almond butter, vanilla protein powder, chia seeds, almond milk, ice cubes and blueberries together until the consistency is smooth.

Nutrition:

Calories: 230,

Carbs: 20 g,

Fat: 8.1 g,

Protein: 21.6 g 72

Salmon and Egg Muffins

Preparation Time: 10 minutes

Cooking Time: 15 minutes

Servings: 2

Ingredients:

- 4 eggs

- 1/3 c. milk

- Salt and pepper

- 1½ oz. smoked salmon

- 1 tbsp. chopped chives

- Green onions, optional

Directions:

2. Preheat the oven to 356 degrees Fahrenheit and grease 6 muffin tin holes with a small amount of olive oil.

3. Place the eggs, milk, and a pinch of salt and pepper into a small bowl and lightly beat to combine.

5. Divide the egg mixture between the 6 muffin holes, then divide the salmon between the muffins and place into each hole, gently pressing down to submerge in the egg mixture, chopped

6. Sprinkle each muffin with chopped chives and place in the oven for about 8-10 minutes or until just set.

7. Leave to cool for about 5 minutes before turning out and storing in an airtight container in the fridge.

Nutrition:

Calories: 93,

Fat: 6g,

Protein: 8g,

Carbs: 1g 74

Stuffed Celery

Preparation Time: 15 Minutes

Cooking Time: 20 Minutes

Servings: 3

Ingredients:

- Olive oil

- 1 clove garlic, minced

- 2 tbsp Pine nuts

- 2 tbsp dry-roasted sunflower seeds

- ¼ cup Italian cheese blend, shredded

- 8 stalks celery leaves

- 1 (8-ounce) fat-free cream cheese

- Cooking spray

Directions:

1. Sauté garlic and pine nuts over a medium setting for the heat until the nuts are golden brown. Cut off the wide base and tops from celery.

2. Remove two thin strips from the round side of the celery to create a flat surface.
3. Mix Italian cheese and cream cheese in a bowl and spread into cut celery stalks.

4. Sprinkle half of the celery pieces with sunflower seeds and a half with the pine nut mixture. Cover mixture and let stand for at least 4 hours before eating.

Nutrition:

Calories: 64

Carbs: 2g

Fat: 6g

Protein: 1g

Butternut Squash Fries

Preparation Time: 5 Minutes

Cooking Time: 10 Minutes

Servings: 2

Ingredients:

- 1 Butternut squash

- 1 tbsp Extra virgin olive oil

- ½ tbsp Grapeseed oil

- 1/8 tsp Sea salt

Directions:

1. Remove seeds from the squash and cut into thin slices. Coat with extra virgin olive oil and grapeseed oil. Add a sprinkle of salt and toss to coat well.

2. Arrange the squash slices onto three baking sheets and bake for 10 minutes until crispy.

Nutrition:

Calories: 40

Carbs: 10g

Fat: 0g

Protein: 1g

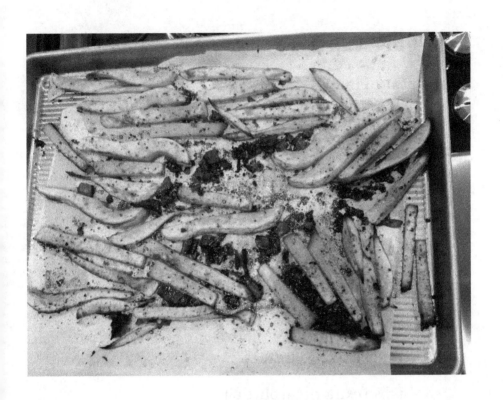

Dried Fig Tapenade

Preparation Time: 5 Minutes

Cooking Time: 0 Minutes

Servings: 1

Ingredients:

- 1 cup Dried figs

- 1 cup Kalamata olives

- ½ cup Water

- 1 tbsp Chopped fresh thyme

- 1 tbsp extra virgin olive oil

- ½ tsp Balsamic vinegar

Directions:

1. Prepare figs in a food processor until well chopped, add water, and continue processing to form a paste.

2. Add olives and pulse until well blended. Add thyme, vinegar, and extra virgin olive oil and pulse until very smooth. Best served with crackers of your choice.

Nutrition:
Calories: 249

Carbs: 64g

Fat: 1g

Protein: 3g

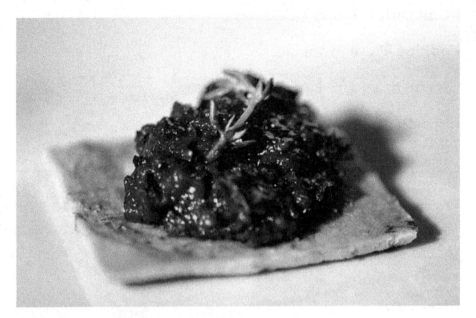

Speedy Sweet Potato Chips

Preparation Time: 15 Minutes

Cooking Time: 0 Minutes

Servings: 4

Ingredients:

- 1 large Sweet potato

- 1 tbsp Extra virgin olive oil

- Salt

Directions:

1. 300°F preheated oven. Slice your potato into nice, thin slices that resemble fries.

2. Toss the potato slices with salt and extra virgin olive oil in a bowl. Bake for about one hour, flipping every 15 minutes until crispy and browned.

Nutrition:

Calories: 150

Carbs: 16g

Fat: 9g

Protein: 1g

Nachos with Hummus (Mediterranean Inspired)

Preparation Time: 15 Minutes

Cooking Time: 20 Minutes

Servings: 4

Ingredients:

- 4 cups salted pita chips

- 1 (8 oz.) red pepper (roasted)

Hummus

- 1 tsp Finely shredded lemon peel

- ¼ cup Chopped pitted Kalamata olives

- ¼ cup crumbled feta cheese

- 1 plum (Roma) tomato, seeded, chopped

- ½ cup chopped cucumber

- 1 tsp Chopped fresh oregano leaves

Directions:

1. 400°F preheated oven. Arrange the pita chips on a heatproof platter and drizzle with hummus.

2. Top with olives, tomato, cucumber, and cheese and bake until warmed through. Sprinkle lemon zest and oregano and enjoy while it's hot.

Nutrition:

Calories: 130

Carbs: 18g

Fat: 5g
Protein: 4g

Hummus and Olive Pita Bread

Preparation Time: 5 Minutes

Cooking Time: 0 Minutes

Servings: 3

Ingredients:

- 7 pita bread cut into 6 wedges each

- 1 (7 ounces) container plain hummus

- 1 tbsp Greek vinaigrette

- ½ cup Chopped pitted Kalamata olives

Directions:

1. Spread the hummus on a serving plate—Mix vinaigrette and olives in a bowl and spoon over the hummus. Enjoy with wedges of pita bread.

Nutrition:

Calories: 225

Carbs: 40g

Fat: 5g

Protein: 9g

Roast Asparagus

Preparation Time: 15 Minutes

Cooking Time: 5 Minutes

Servings: 4

Ingredients:

- 1 tbsp Extra virgin olive oil (1 tablespoon)

- 1 medium lemon

- ½ tsp Freshly grated nutmeg

- ½ tsp black pepper

- ½ tsp Kosher salt

Directions:

1. Warm the oven to 500°F. Put the asparagus on an aluminum foil and drizzle with extra virgin olive oil, and toss until well coated.

2. Roast the asparagus in the oven for about five minutes; toss and continue roasting until browned. Sprinkle the roasted asparagus with nutmeg, salt, zest, and pepper.

Nutrition:

Calories: 123

Carbs: 5g

Fat: 11g

Protein: 3g

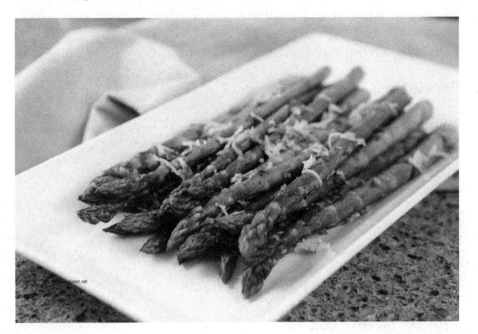

Chicken Kale Wraps

Preparation Time: 10 Minutes

Cooking Time: 10 Minutes

Servings: 4

Ingredients:
- 4 kale leaves
- 4 oz chicken fillet
- ½ apple
- 1 tablespoon butter
- ¼ teaspoon chili pepper
- ¾ teaspoon salt
- 1 tablespoon lemon juice
- ¾ teaspoon dried thyme

Directions:

1. Chop the chicken fillet into small cubes. Then mix up the chicken with chili pepper and salt.

2. Heat butter in the skillet. Add chicken cubes. Roast them for 4 minutes.
3. Meanwhile, chop the apple into small cubes and add to the chicken. Mix up well.
4. Sprinkle the ingredients with lemon juice and dried thyme. Cook them for 5 minutes over medium-high heat.

5. Fill the kale leaves with the hot chicken mixture and wrap.

Nutrition:

Calories 106

Fat 5.1

Fiber 1.1

Carbs 6.3

Protein 9

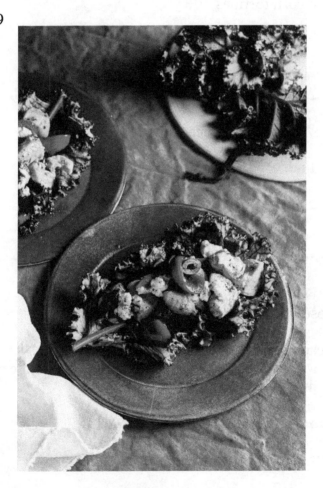

Tomato Triangles

Preparation Time: 10 Minutes

Cooking Time: 0 Minutes

Servings: 6

Ingredients:

- 6 corn tortillas

- 1 tablespoon cream cheese
- 1 tablespoon ricotta cheese
- ½ teaspoon minced garlic
- 1 tablespoon fresh dill, chopped
- 2 tomatoes, sliced

Directions:

1. Cut every tortilla into 2 triangles. Then mix up cream cheese, ricotta cheese, minced garlic, and dill.
2. Spread 6 triangles with cream cheese mixture.
3. Then place the sliced tomato on them and cover with remaining tortilla triangles. Serve.

Nutrition:

Calories 71

Fat 1.6

Fiber 2.1

Carbs 12.8

Protein 2.3

Zaatar Fries

Preparation Time: 10 Minutes

Cooking Time: 35 Minutes

Servings: 5
Ingredients:

- 1 teaspoon Zaatar spices

- 3 sweet potatoes

- 1 tablespoon dried dill

- 1 teaspoon salt

- 3 teaspoons sunflower oil

- ½ teaspoon paprika

Directions:

1. Pour water into the crockpot. Cut the sweet potatoes into fries.

2. Line the baking tray with parchment. Place the layer of the sweet potato in the tray.
3. Sprinkle the vegetables with dried dill, salt, and paprika. Then sprinkle sweet potatoes with Za'atar and mix up well with the help of the fingertips.
4. Sprinkle the sweet potato fries with sunflower oil—Preheat the oven to 375F.
5. Bake the sweet potato fries within 35 minutes. Stir the fries every 10 minutes.

Nutrition:

Calories 28

Fat 2.9

Fiber 0.2

Carbs 0.6

Protein 0.2

Summertime Vegetable Chicken Wraps

Preparation Time: 15 Minutes

Cooking Time: 0 Minutes

Servings: 4

Ingredients:

- 2 cups cooked chicken, chopped

- ½ English cucumbers, diced

- ½ red bell pepper, diced

- ½ cup carrot, shredded

- 1 scallion, white and green parts, chopped

- ¼ cup plain Greek yogurt

- 1 tablespoon freshly squeezed lemon juice

- ½ teaspoon fresh thyme, chopped

- Pinch of salt

- Pinch of ground black pepper

- 4 multigrain tortillas

Directions:

1. Take a medium bowl and mix in chicken, red bell pepper, cucumber, carrot, yogurt, scallion, lemon juice, thyme, sea salt and pepper.

2. Mix well.
3. Spoon one quarter of chicken mix into the middle of the tortilla and fold the opposite ends of the tortilla over the filling.
4. Roll the tortilla from the side to create a snug pocket.
5. Repeat with the remaining ingredients and serve.
6. Enjoy!

Nutrition:

Calories: 278
Fat: 4g

Carbohydrates: 28g

Protein: 27g

Premium Roasted Baby Potatoes

Preparation Time: 10 Minutes

Cooking Time: 35 Minutes

Servings: 4

Ingredients:

- 2 pounds new yellow potatoes, scrubbed and cut into wedges

- 2 tablespoons extra virgin olive oil

- 2 teaspoons fresh rosemary, chopped

- 1 teaspoon garlic powder

- 1 teaspoon sweet paprika

- ½ teaspoon sea salt

- ½ teaspoon freshly ground black pepper

Directions:

1. Pre-heat your oven to 400 degrees Fahrenheit.
2. Take a large bowl and add potatoes, olive oil, garlic, rosemary, paprika, sea salt and pepper.
3. Spread potatoes in single layer on baking sheet and bake for 35 minutes.
4. Serve and enjoy!

Nutrition:

Calories: 225

Fat: 7g

Carbohydrates: 37g

Protein: 5g

Tomato and Cherry Linguine

Preparation Time: 10 Minutes

Cooking Time: 15 Minutes

Servings: 4

Ingredients:

- 2 pounds cherry tomatoes

- 3 tablespoons extra virgin olive oil

- 2 tablespoons balsamic vinegar

- 2 teaspoons garlic, minced

- Pinch of fresh ground black pepper

- ¾ pound whole-wheat linguine pasta

- 1 tablespoon fresh oregano, chopped

- ¼ cup feta cheese, crumbled

Directions:

1. Pre-heat your oven to 350 degrees Fahrenheit.

2. Take a large bowl and add cherry tomatoes, 2 tablespoons olive oil, balsamic vinegar, garlic, pepper and toss.

3. Spread tomatoes evenly on baking sheet and roast for 15 minutes.

4. While the tomatoes are roasting, cook the pasta according to the package instructions and drain the paste into a large bowl.
5. Toss pasta with 1 tablespoon olive oil.
6. Add roasted tomatoes (with juice) and toss.
7. Serve with topping of oregano and feta cheese.

8. Enjoy!

Nutrition:

Calories: 397

Fat: 15g

Carbohydrates: 55g

Protein: 13g

Mediterranean Zucchini Mushroom Pasta

Preparation Time: 10 Minutes

Cooking Time: 10 Minutes

Servings: 4

Ingredients:

- ½ pound pasta

- 2 tablespoons olive oil

- 6 garlic cloves, crushed

- 1 teaspoon red chili

- 2 spring onions, sliced

- 3 teaspoons rosemary

- 1 large zucchini, cut in half

- 5 large portabella mushrooms

- 1 can tomatoes

- 4 tablespoons Parmesan cheese

- Fresh ground black pepper

Directions:

1. Cook the pasta.

2. Take a large-sized frying pan and place it over medium heat.
3. Add oil and allow the oil to heat up.
4. Add garlic, onion and chili and sauté for a few minutes until golden.
5. Add zucchini, rosemary and mushroom and sauté for a few minutes.
6. Increase the heat to medium-high and add tinned tomatoes to the sauce until thick.

7. Drain your boiled pasta and transfer to serving platter.
8. Pour the tomato mix on top and mix using tongs.
9. Garnish with Parmesan and freshly ground black pepper.
10. Enjoy!

Nutrition:

Calories: 361

Fat: 12g

Carbohydrates: 47g

Protein: 14g

Lemon and Garlic Fettucine

Preparation Time: 5 Minutes

Cooking Time: 15 Minutes

Servings: 5

Ingredients:

-
  8 ounces of whole wheat fettuccine
- 4 tablespoons of extra virgin olive oil

- 4 cloves of minced garlic

- 1 cup of fresh breadcrumbs

- ¼ cup of lemon juice

- 1 teaspoon of freshly ground pepper

- ½ teaspoon of salt

- 2 cans of 4 ounce boneless and skinless sardines (dipped in tomato sauce)

- ½ cup of chopped up fresh parsley

- ¼ cup of finely shredded Parmesan cheese

Directions:

1. Take a large-sized pot and bring water to a boil.

2. Cook pasta for 10 minutes until Al Dente.
3. Take a small-sized skillet and place it over medium heat.
4. Add 2 tablespoons of oil and allow it to heat up.

5. Add garlic and cook for 20 seconds.
6. Transfer the garlic to a medium-sized bowl
7. Add breadcrumbs to the hot skillet and cook for 5-6 minutes until golden
8. Whisk in lemon juice, pepper and salt into the garlic bowl
9. Add pasta to the bowl (with garlic) and sardines, parsley and Parmesan
10. Stir well and sprinkle bread crumbs
11. Enjoy!

Nutrition:

Calories: 480

Fat: 21g

Carbohydrates: 53g

Protein: 23g

Roasted Broccoli with Parmesan

Preparation Time: 10 Minutes

Cooking Time: 10 Minutes

Servings: 4

Ingredients:

- 2 head broccolis, cut into florets

- 2 tablespoons extra-virgin olive oil

- 2 teaspoons garlic, minced

- Zest of 1 lemon

- Pinch of salt

- ½ cup Parmesan cheese, grated

Directions:

1. Pre-heat your oven to 400 degrees Fahrenheit.

2. Take a large bowl and add broccoli with 2 tablespoons olive oil, lemon zest, garlic, lemon juice and salt.

3. Spread mix on the baking sheet in single layer and sprinkle with Parmesan cheese.
4. Bake for 10 minutes until tender.
5. Transfer broccoli to serving the dish.
6. Serve and enjoy!

Nutrition:

Calories: 154

Fat: 11g

Carbohydrates: 10g
Protein: 9g

Spinach and Feta Bread

Preparation Time: 10 Minutes

Cooking Time: 12 Minutes

Servings: 6

Ingredients:

- 6 ounces of sun-dried tomato pesto

- 6 pieces of 6-inch whole wheat pita bread

- 2 chopped up Roma plum tomatoes

- 1 bunch of rinsed and chopped spinach

- 4 sliced fresh mushrooms

- ½ cup of crumbled feta cheese

- 2 tablespoons of grated Parmesan cheese

- 3 tablespoons of olive oil

- Ground black pepper as needed

Directions:

1. Pre-heat your oven to 350 degrees Fahrenheit.

2. Spread your tomato pesto onto one side of your pita bread and place on your baking sheet (with the pesto side up).
3. Top up the pitas with spinach, tomatoes, feta cheese, mushrooms and Parmesan cheese.
4. Drizzle with some olive oil and season nicely with pepper.

5. Bake in your oven for around 12 minutes until the breads are crispy.
6. Cut up the pita into quarters and serve!

Nutrition:

Calories: 350

Fat: 17g

Carbohydrates: 41g

Protein:11g

Quick Zucchini Bowl

Preparation Time: 10 Minutes

Cooking Time: 10 Minutes

Servings: 4

Ingredients:

- ½ pound of pasta

- 2 tablespoons of olive oil

- 6 crushed garlic cloves

- 1 teaspoon of red chili

- 2 finely sliced spring onions

- 3 teaspoons of chopped rosemary

- 1 large zucchini cut up in half, lengthways and sliced

- 5 large portabella mushrooms

- 1 can of tomatoes

- 4 tablespoons of Parmesan cheese

- Fresh ground black pepper

Directions:

1. Cook the pasta.

3. Take a large-sized frying pan and place over medium heat.

4. Add oil and allow the oil to heat up.

5. Add garlic, onion and chili and sauté for a few minutes until golden.
6. Add zucchini, rosemary and mushroom and sauté for a few minutes.
7. Increase the heat to medium-high and add tinned tomatoes to the sauce until thick.

8. Drain your boiled pasta and transfer to a serving platter.
9. Pour the tomato mix on top and mix using tongs.
10. Garnish with Parmesan cheese and freshly ground black pepper.
11. Enjoy!

Nutrition:

Calories: 361

Fat: 12g

Carbohydrates: 47g

Protein: 14g

Healthy Basil Platter

Preparation Time: 25 Minutes

Cooking Time: 15 Minutes

Servings: 4

Ingredients:

- 2 pieces of red pepper seeded and cut up into chunks

- 2 pieces of red onion cut up into wedges

- 2 mild red chilies, diced and seeded

- 3 coarsely chopped garlic cloves

- 1 teaspoon of golden caster sugar

- 2 tablespoons of olive oil (plus additional for serving)

- 2 pounds of small ripe tomatoes quartered up

- 12 ounces of dried pasta

- Just a handful of basil leaves

- 2 tablespoons of grated Parmesan

Directions:

1. Pre-heat the oven to 392 degrees Fahrenheit.

2. Take a large-sized roasting tin and scatter pepper, red onion, garlic and chilies.

3. Sprinkle sugar on top.
4. Drizzle olive oil then season with pepper and salt.
5. Roast the veggies in your oven for 15 minutes.
6. Take a large-sized pan and cook the pasta in boiling, salted water until Al Dente.

7. Drain them.
8. Remove the veggies from the oven and tip in the pasta into the veggies.
9. Toss well and tear basil leaves on top.
10. Sprinkle Parmesan and enjoy!

Nutrition:

Calories: 452

Fat: 8g

Carbohydrates: 88g

Protein: 14g

Tomato Bruschetta

Preparation Time: 10 Minutes

Cooking Time: 10 Minutes
Servings: 6

Ingredients:

- 1 baguette, sliced

- 1/3 cup basil, chopped

- 6 tomatoes, cubed

- 2 garlic cloves, minced

- A pinch of salt and black pepper

- 1 teaspoon olive oil

- 1 tablespoon balsamic vinegar

- ½ teaspoon garlic powder

- Cooking spray

Directions:

1. Arrange the baguette slices in the baking sheet lined with parchment paper, grease them with cooking spray and bake at 400 degrees F for 10 minutes.

2. In a bowl, mix the tomatoes with the basil and the remaining ingredients, toss well and leave aside for 10 minutes.
3. Divide the tomato mix on each baguette slice, arrange them all on a platter and serve.

Nutrition:

Calories: 162,

Fat: 4,

Fiber: 7,

Carbs: 29,

Protein: 4

Artichoke Flatbread

Preparation Time: 10 Minutes

Cooking Time: 15 Minutes

Servings: 4

Ingredients:

- 5 tablespoons olive oil

- 2 garlic cloves, minced

- 2 tablespoons parsley, chopped

- 2 round whole wheat flatbreads

- 4 tablespoons parmesan, grated

- ½ cup mozzarella cheese, grated

- 14 ounces canned artichokes, drained and quartered

- 1 cup baby spinach, chopped

- ½ cup cherry tomatoes, halved

- ½ teaspoon basil, dried

- Salt and black pepper to the taste

Directions:

1. In a bowl, mix the parsley with the garlic and 4 tablespoons oil, whisk well and spread this over the flatbreads.

2. Sprinkle the mozzarella and half of the parmesan.
3. In a bowl, mix the artichokes with the spinach, tomatoes, basil, salt, pepper and the rest of the oil, toss and divide over the flatbreads as well.
4. Sprinkle the remaining of the parmesan on top, arrange the flatbreads on a baking sheet lined with parchment paper and bake at 425 degrees F for 15 minutes.
5. Serve.

Nutrition:

Calories: 223,

Fat: 11.2,

Fiber: 5.34,

Carbs: 15.5,

Protein: 7.4

Red Pepper Tapenade

Preparation Time: 10 Minutes

Cooking Time: 0 Minutes

Servings: 4

Ingredients:

- 7 ounces roasted red peppers, chopped

- ½ cup parmesan, grated

- 1/3 cup parsley, chopped

- 14 ounces canned artichokes, drained and chopped

- 3 tablespoons olive oil

- ¼ cup capers, drained

- 1 and ½ tablespoons lemon juice

- 2 garlic cloves, minced

Directions:

1. In your blender, combine the red peppers with the parmesan and the rest of the ingredients and pulse well.

2. Divide into cups and serve.

Nutrition:

Calories: 200,

Fat: 5.6,

Fiber: 4.5,

Carbs: 12.4,

Protein: 4.6

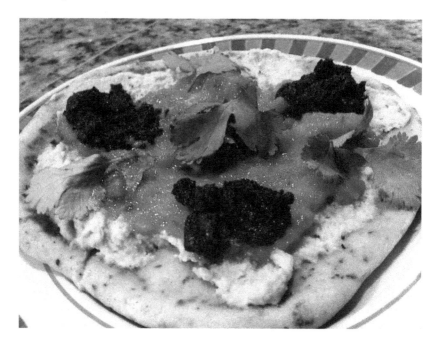

Coriander Falafel

Preparation Time: 10 Minutes

Cooking Time: 10 Minutes

Servings: 8

Ingredients:

- 1 cup canned garbanzo beans, drained and rinsed

- 1 bunch parsley leaves

- 1 yellow onion, chopped

- 5 garlic cloves, minced

- 1 teaspoon coriander, ground

- A pinch of salt and black pepper

- ¼ teaspoon cayenne pepper

- ¼ teaspoon baking soda

- ¼ teaspoon cumin powder

- 1 teaspoon lemon juice

- 3 tablespoons tapioca flour
- Olive oil for frying

Directions:

1. In your food processor, combine the beans with the parsley, onion and the rest the ingredients except the oil and the flour and pulse well.

2. Transfer the mix to a bowl, add the flour, stir well, shape 16 balls out of this mix and flatten them a bit.

3. Heat up a pan with some oil over medium-high heat, add the falafels, cook them for 5 minutes on each side, transfer to paper towels, drain excess grease, arrange them on a platter and serve as an appetizer.

Nutrition:

Calories: 112,

Fat: 6.2,

Fiber: 2,

Carbs: 12.3,

Protein: 3.1

Chapter 9: Snacks Recipes

Cinnamon and Hemp Seed Coffee Shake

Preparation Time: 5 Minutes

Cooking Time: 0 Minutes

Servings: 1

Ingredients:

- 1 ½ frozen bananas, sliced into coins

- 1/8 teaspoon ground cinnamon

- 2 tablespoons hemp seeds

- 1 tablespoon maple syrup

- ¼ teaspoon vanilla extract, unsweetened

- 1 cup regular coffee, cooled

- ¼ cup almond milk, unsweetened

- ½ cup of ice cubes

Directions:

1. Pour milk into a blender, add vanilla, cinnamon, and hemp seeds and then pulse until smooth.

2. Add banana, pour in the coffee, and then pulse until smooth.
3. Add ice, blend until well combined, blend in maple syrup and then serve.

Nutrition:

Calories: 410 Cal;

Fat: 19.5 g;

Protein: 4.9 g;

Carbs: 60.8 g;

Fiber: 6.8 g

Green Smoothie

Preparation Time: 5 Minutes

Cooking Time: 0 Minutes

Servings: 1

Ingredients:

- ½ cup strawberries, frozen

- 4 leaves of kale

- ¼ of a medium banana

- 2 Medjool dates, pitted

- 1 tablespoon flax seed

- ¼ cup pumpkin seeds, hulled

- 1 cup of water

Directions:

1. Place all the ingredients in the jar of a food processor or blender and then cover it with the lid.

2. Pulse until smooth and then serve.

Nutrition:

Calories: 204 Cal;

Fat: 1.1 g;

Protein: 6.5 g;

Carbs: 48 g;
Fiber: 8.3 g

Strawberry and Banana Smoothie

Preparation Time: 5 Minutes

Cooking Time: 0 Minutes

Servings: 1

Ingredients:

- 1 cup sliced banana, frozen

- 2 tablespoons chia seeds

- 2 cups strawberries, frozen

- 2 teaspoons honey

- ¼ teaspoon vanilla extract, unsweetened

- 6 ounces coconut yogurt

- 1 cup almond milk, unsweetened

Directions:

1. Place all the ingredients in the jar of a food processor or blender and then cover it with the lid.

2. Pulse until smooth and then serve.

Nutrition:

Calories: 114 Cal;

Fat: 2.1 g;

Protein: 3.7 g;

Carbs: 22.3 g;

Fiber: 3.8 g

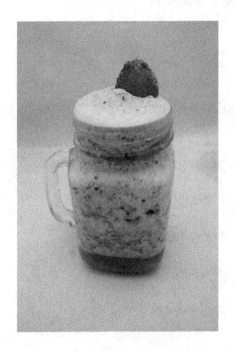

Orange Smoothie

Preparation Time: 5 Minutes

Cooking Time: 0 Minutes

Servings: 1

Ingredients:

- 1 cup slices of oranges

- ½ teaspoon grated ginger
- 1 cup of mango pieces
- 1 cup of coconut water
- 1 cup chopped strawberries
- 1 cup crushed ice

Directions:

1. Place all the ingredients in the jar of a food processor or blender and then cover it with the lid.

2. Pulse until smooth and then serve.

Nutrition:

Calories: 198.7 Cal;

Fat: 1.2 g;

Protein: 6.1 g;

Carbs: 34.3 g;

Fiber: 0 g

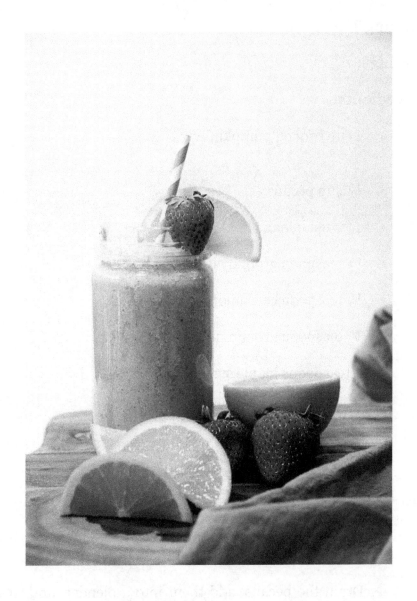

Pumpkin Chai Smoothie

Preparation Time: 5 Minutes

Cooking Time: 0 Minutes

Servings: 1

Ingredients:

- 1 cup cooked pumpkin

- ¼ cup pecans

- 1 frozen banana

- ¼ teaspoon ground cinnamon

- ¼ teaspoon cardamom

- ¼ teaspoon ground nutmeg

- 2 teaspoons maple syrup

- 1 cup of water, cold

- ½ cup of ice cubes

Directions:

1. Place pecans in a small bowl, cover with water, and then let them soak for 10 minutes.

2. Drain the pecans, add them into a blender, and then add the remaining ingredients.
3. Pulse for 1 minute until smooth, and then serve.

Nutrition:

Calories: 157.5 Cal;

Fat: 3.8 g;

Protein: 3 g;

Carbs: 32.3 g;

Fiber: 4.5 g

Banana Shake

Preparation Time: 5 Minutes

Cooking Time: 0 Minutes

Servings: 1

Ingredients:

- 3 medium frozen bananas

- 1 tablespoon cocoa powder, unsweetened

- 1 teaspoon shredded coconut

- 1 tablespoon maple syrup

- 1 tablespoon peanut butter

- 1 teaspoon vanilla extract, unsweetened

- 2 cups of coconut water

- 1 cup of ice cubes

Directions:

1. Add banana in a food processor, add maple syrup and vanilla, pour in water and then add ice.

2. Pulse until smooth and then pour half of the smoothie into a glass.
3. Add butter and cocoa powder into the blender, pulse until smooth, and then add to the smoothie glass.

4. Sprinkle coconut over the smoothie and then serve.

Nutrition:

Calories: 301 Cal;

Fat: 9.3 g;
Protein: 6.8 g;

Carbs: 49 g;

Fiber: 1.9 g

Green Honeydew Smoothie

Preparation Time: 5 Minutes

Cooking Time: 15 Minutes

Servings: 4

Ingredients:

- 1 large banana

- 6 large leaves of basil

- ½ cup frozen pineapple

- 1 teaspoon lime juice

- 1 cup pieces of honeydew melon

- 1 teaspoon green tea matcha powder

- ¼ cup almond milk, unsweetened

Directions:

1. Place all the ingredients in the jar of a food processor or blender and then cover it with the lid.

2. Pulse until smooth and then serve.

Nutrition:

Calories: 223.5 Cal;

Fat: 2.7 g;

Protein: 20.1 g;

Carbs: 32.7 g;

Fiber: 5.2 g

Summer Salsa

Preparation Time: 5 Minutes

Cooking Time: 15 Minutes

Servings: 8

Ingredients:

- 1 cup cherry tomatoes, chopped

- ¼ cup chopped cilantro
- 2 tablespoons chopped red onion
- 1 teaspoon minced garlic
- 1 small jalapeno, deseeded, chopped
- ½ of a lime, juiced
- 1/8 teaspoon salt
- 1 tablespoon olive oil

Directions:

1. Place all the ingredients in the jar of a food processor or blender except for cilantro and then cover with its lid.
2. Pulse until smooth and then pulse in cilantro until evenly mixed.
3. Tip the salsa into a bowl and then serve with vegetable sticks.

Nutrition:

Calories: 51 Cal;
Fat: 0.1 g;

Protein: 1.7 g;

Carbs: 11.4 g;

Fiber: 3.1 g

Red Salsa

Preparation Time: 35 Minutes

Cooking Time: 15 Minutes

Servings: 8

Ingredients:

- 4 Roma tomatoes, halved

- ¼ cup chopped cilantro

- 1 jalapeno pepper, deseeded, halved

- ½ of a medium white onion, peeled, cut into quarters

- 3 cloves of garlic, peeled

- ½ teaspoon salt

- 1 tablespoon brown sugar

- 1 teaspoon apple cider vinegar

Directions:

1. Switch on the oven, then set it to 425 degrees F and let it preheat.

2. Meanwhile, take a baking sheet, line it with foil, and then spread tomato, jalapeno pepper, onion, and garlic.

3. Bake the vegetables for 15 minutes until vegetables have cooked and begin to brown and then let the vegetables cool for 3 minutes.

4. Transfer the roasted vegetables into a blender, add remaining ingredients and then pulse until smooth.

5. Tip the salsa into a medium bowl and then chill it for 30 minutes before serving with vegetable sticks.

Nutrition:

Calories: 240 Cal;

Fat: 0 g;

Protein: 0 g;

Carbs: 48 g;

Fiber: 16 g

Pinto Bean Dip

Preparation Time: 5 Minutes

Cooking Time: 0 Minutes

Servings: 4

Ingredients:

- 15 ounces canned pinto beans

- 1 jalapeno pepper

- 2 teaspoons ground cumin

- 3 tablespoons nutritional yeast

- 1/3 cup basil salsa

Directions:

1. Place all the ingredients in a food processor, cover with the lid, and then pulse until smooth.

2. Tip the dip in a bowl and then serve with vegetable slices.

Nutrition:

Calories: 360 Cal;

Fat: 0 g;

Protein: 24 g;

Carbs: 72 g;

Fiber: 24 g

Smoky Red Pepper Hummus

Preparation Time: 5 Minutes

Cooking Time: 0 Minutes

Servings: 4

Ingredients:

- ¼ cup roasted red peppers

- 1 cup cooked chickpeas

- 1/8 teaspoon garlic powder

- ½ teaspoon salt

- 1/8 teaspoon ground black pepper

- ¼ teaspoon ground cumin

- ¼ teaspoon red chili powder

- 1 tablespoon Tahini

- 2 tablespoons water

Directions:

1. Place all the ingredients in the jar of the food processor and then pulse until smooth.

2. Tip the hummus in a bowl and then serve with vegetable slices.

Nutrition:

Calories: 489 Cal;

Fat: 30 g;

Protein: 9 g;

Carbs: 15 g;

Fiber: 6 g

Spinach Dip

Preparation Time: 20 Minutes

Cooking Time: 5 Minutes

Servings: 8

Ingredients:

- ¾ cup cashews

- 3.5 ounces soft tofu

- 6 ounces of spinach leaves

- 1 medium white onion, peeled, diced

- 2 teaspoons minced garlic

- ½ teaspoon salt

- 3 tablespoons olive oil

Directions:

1. Place cashews in a bowl, cover with hot water, and then let them soak for 15 minutes.
2. After 15 minutes, drain the cashews and then set aside until required.

3. Take a medium skillet pan, add oil to it and then place the pan over medium heat.
4. Add onion, cook for 3 to 5 minutes until tender, stir in garlic and then continue cooking for 30 seconds until fragrant.

5. Spoon the onion mixture into a blender, add remaining ingredients and then pulse until smooth.

6. Tip the dip into a bowl and then serve with chips.

Nutrition:

Calories: 134.6 Cal;

Fat: 8.6 g;

Protein: 10 g;

Carbs: 6.3 g;

Fiber: 1.4 g

Tomatillo Salsa

Preparation Time: 5 Minutes

Cooking Time: 20 Minutes

Servings: 8

Ingredients:

- 5 medium tomatillos, chopped

- 3 cloves of garlic, peeled, chopped
- 3 Roma tomatoes, chopped
- 1 jalapeno, chopped
- ½ of a medium red onion, peeled, chopped
- 1 Anaheim chili
- 2 teaspoons salt
- 1 teaspoon ground cumin
- 1 lime, juiced
- ¼ cup cilantro leaves
- ¾ cup of water

Directions:

1. Take a medium pot, place it over medium heat, pour in water, and then add onion, tomatoes, tomatillo, jalapeno, and Anaheim chili.

2. Sauté the vegetables for 15 minutes, remove the pot from heat, add cilantro and lime juice and then stir in salt.
3. Remove pot from heat and then pulse by using an immersion blender until smooth.
4. Serve the salsa with chips.

Nutrition:

Calories: 317.4 Cal;

Fat: 0 g;

Protein: 16 g;

Carbs: 64 g;

Fiber: 16 g

Arugula Pesto Couscous

Preparation Time: 10 Minutes

Cooking Time: 20 Minutes

Servings: 4
Ingredients:

- 8 ounces Israeli couscous

- 3 large tomatoes, chopped

- 3 cups arugula leaves

- ½ cup parsley leaves

- 6 cloves of garlic, peeled

- ½ cup walnuts

- ¾ teaspoon salt

- 1 cup and 1 tablespoon olive oil

- 2 cups vegetable broth

Directions:

1. Take a medium saucepan, place it over medium-high heat, add 1 tablespoon oil and then let it heat.

2. Add couscous, stir until mixed, and then cook for 4 minutes until fragrant and toasted.
3. Pour in the broth, stir until mixed, bring it to a boil, switch heat to medium level and then simmer for 12

minutes until the couscous has absorbed all the liquid and turn tender.

4. When done, remove the pan from heat, fluff it with a fork, and then set aside until required.
5. While couscous cooks, prepare the pesto, and for this, place walnuts in a blender, add garlic, and then pulse until nuts have broken.
6. Add arugula, parsley, and salt, pulse until well combined, and then blend in oil until smooth.
7. Transfer couscous to a salad bowl, add tomatoes and prepared pesto, and then toss until mixed.

8. Serve straight away.

Nutrition:

Calories: 73 Cal;

Fat: 4 g;

Protein: 2 g;

Carbs: 8 g;

Fiber: 2 g

Oatmeal and Raisin Balls

Preparation Time: 40 Minutes

Cooking Time: 0 Minutes

Servings: 4

Ingredients:

- 1 cup rolled oats

- ¼ cup raisins
- ½ cup peanut butter

Directions:

1. Place oats in a large bowl, add raisins and peanut butter, and then stir until well combined.

2. Shape the mixture into twelve balls, 1 tablespoon of mixture per ball, and then arrange the balls on a baking sheet.
3. Place the baking sheet into the freezer for 30 minutes until firm and then serve.

Nutrition:

Calories: 135 Cal;

Fat: 6 g;

Protein: 8 g;

Carbs: 13 g;
Fiber: 4 g

Nacho Cheese

Preparation Time: 10 Minutes

Cooking Time: 15 Minutes

Servings: 4

Ingredients:

- 1 cup chopped carrots

- ½ teaspoon onion powder

- 2 cups peeled and chopped potatoes

- ½ teaspoon garlic powder

- 1 teaspoon salt

- ½ cup nutritional yeast

- 1 tablespoon lemon juice

- ¼ cup of salsa

- ½ cup of water

Directions:

1. Take a medium pot, place carrots and potato in it, cover with water and then place the pot over medium-high heat.

2. Boil the vegetables for 10 minutes, drain them, and then transfer into a blender.

3. Add remaining ingredients and then pulse until smooth.
4. Tip the cheese into a bowl and then serve with vegetable slices.

Nutrition:

Calories: 611.7 Cal;

Fat: 17.2 g;

Protein: 32.1 g;

Carbs: 62.1 g;

Fiber: 12.1 g

Pico de Gallo

Preparation Time: 5 Minutes

Cooking Time: 0 Minutes

Servings: 6

Ingredients:

- ½ of a medium red onion, peeled, chopped

- 2 cups diced tomato

- ½ cup chopped cilantro

- 1 jalapeno pepper, minced

- 1/8 teaspoon salt

- ¼ teaspoon ground black pepper

- ½ of a lime, juiced

- 1 teaspoon olive oil

Directions:

1. Take a large bowl, place all the ingredients in it and then stir until well mixed.

2. Serve the Pico de Gallo with chips.

Nutrition:

Calories: 790 Cal;
Fat: 6.4 g;

Protein: 25.6 g;

Carbs: 195.2 g;

Fiber: 35.2 g

Moroccan-Style Couscous with Chickpeas

Preparation Time: 5 minutes

Cooking Time: 18 minutes

Servings: 2
Ingredients

- Extra-virgin olive oil – ¼ cup, extra for serving

- Couscous – 1 ½ cups

- Peeled and chopped fine carrots – 2

- Chopped fine onion – 1

- Salt and pepper

- Garlic – 3 cloves, minced

- Ground coriander – 1 tsp.

- Ground ginger - tsp.

- Ground anise seed – ¼ tsp.

- Chicken broth – 1 ¾ cups

- Chickpeas - 1 (15-ounce) can, rinsed

- Frozen peas – 1 ½ cups

- Chopped fresh parsley or cilantro – ½ cup

- Lemon wedges

Directions

1. Heat 2 tbsp. oil in a skillet over medium heat.

2. Add the couscous and cook for 3 to 5 minutes, or until just beginning to brown.
3. Transfer to a bowl and clean the skillet.
4. Heat remaining 2 tbsp. oil in the skillet and add the onion, carrots, and 1 tsp. salt.
5. Cook for 5 to 7 minutes, or until softened.
6. Stir in anise, ginger, coriander, and garlic. Cook until fragrant (about 30 seconds).
7. Stir in the chickpeas and broth and bring to simmer.
8. Stir in the couscous and peas. Cover and remove from the heat. Set aside for 7 minutes, or until the couscous is tender.
9. Add the parsley to the couscous and fluff with a fork to combine.
10. Drizzle with extra oil and season with salt and pepper.
11. Serve with lemon wedges.

Nutrition

Calories: 649

Fat: 14.2g

Carb: 102.8g

Protein: 30.1g

Vegetarian Paella with Green Beans and Chickpeas

Preparation Time: 10 minutes

Cooking Time: 35 minutes

Servings: 2

Ingredients

- Pinch of saffron
- Vegetable broth – 3 cups
- Olive oil – 1 tbsp.
- Yellow onion – 1 large, diced
- Garlic – 4 cloves, sliced
- Red bell pepper – 1, diced
- Crushed tomatoes – ¾ cup, fresh or canned
- Tomato paste – 2 tbsp.
- Hot paprika – 1 ½ tsp.
- Salt – 1 tsp.
- Freshly ground black pepper – ½ tsp.
-
  Green beans – 1 ½ cups, trimmed and halved
- Chickpeas – 1 (15-ounce) can, drained and rinsed

  Short-grain white rice – 1 cup

•

- Lemon – 1, cut into wedges

Directions

1. Mix the saffron threads with 3 tbsp. warm water in a small bowl.

2. In a saucepan, bring the water to a simmer over medium heat. Lower the heat to low and let the broth simmer.
3. Heat the oil in a skillet over medium heat. Add the onion and stir-fry for 5 minutes.
4. Add the bell pepper and garlic and stir-fry for 7 minutes or until pepper is softened.
5. Stir in the saffron-water mixture, salt, pepper, paprika, tomato paste, and tomatoes.
6. Add the rice, chickpeas, and green beans. Add the warm broth and bring to a boil.
7. Lower the heat and simmer uncovered for 20 minutes.
8. Serve hot, garnished with lemon wedges.

Nutrition

Calories: 709

Fat: 12g

Carb: 121g

Protein: 33g

Garlic Prawns with Tomatoes and Basil

Preparation Time: 10 minutes

Cooking Time: 10 minutes

Servings: 2

Ingredients

- Olive oil – 2 tbsp.

- Prawns – 1 ¼ pounds, peeled and deveined

- Garlic – 3 cloves, minced

- Crushed red pepper flakes – 1/8 tsp.

- Dry white wine – ¾ cup

- Grape tomatoes – 1 ½ cups

- Finely chopped fresh basil – ¼ cup, plus more for garnish

- Salt – ¾ tsp.

- Ground black pepper – ½ tsp.

Directions

1. In a skillet, heat oil over medium-high heat. Add the prawns and cook for 1 minute, or until just cooked through. Transfer to a plate.

2. Add the red pepper flakes, and garlic to the oil in the pan and cook, stirring, for 30 seconds. Stir in the wine and cook until it's reduced by about half.
3. Add the tomatoes and stir-fry until tomatoes begin to break down (about 3 to 4 minutes). Stir in the reserved shrimp, salt, pepper, and basil. Cook for 1 to 2 minutes more.
4. Serve garnished with the remaining basil.

Nutrition

Calories: 282

Fat: 10g

Carb: 7g

Protein: 33g

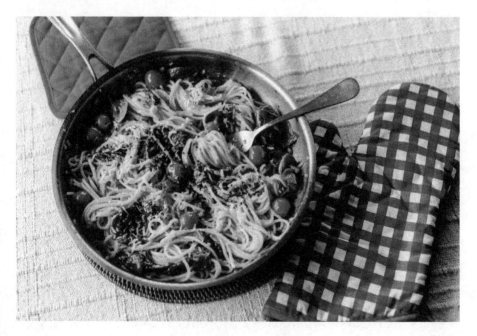

Stuffed Calamari in Tomato Sauce

Preparation Time: 10 minutes

Cooking Time: 25 minutes

Servings: 2

Ingredients

- Olive oil – ½ cup, plus 3 tbsp. divided
- Large onions - 2, finely chopped
- Garlic – 4 cloves, finely chopped
- Grated Pecorino Romano – 1 cup, plus ¼ cup, divided
- Chopped flat-leaf parsley – ½ cup, plus ¼ cup, divided
- Breadcrumbs – 6 cups
- Raisins – 1 cup
- Large squid tubes – 12, cleaned
- Toothpicks – 12
- For the tomato sauce
- Olive oil – 2 tbsp.
- Garlic – 4 cloves, chopped
- Crushed tomatoes – 2 (28-ounce) cans
- Finely chopped basil – ½ cup

- Salt – 1 tsp.

- Pepper – 1 tsp.

Directions

1. Combine the saffron threads with 2 tbsp. of warm water.

2. In a Dutch oven, heat ½ cup of olive oil. Add the onions and ½ tsp. of salt and stir-fry for 5 minutes. Add the tomato paste and cook for 1 minute more.

3. Add the wine and bring to a boil. Add the fish broth and soaked saffron and bring back to a boil. Lower the heat to low and simmer, uncovered, for 10 minutes.

4. Meanwhile, in a food processor, combine the bread and garlic, and process until ground.

5. Add the remaining ¼ cup olive oil and ½ tsp. salt and pulse just to mix.

6. Add the fish to the pot, cover, and cook until the fish is just cooked through, about 6 minutes. Stir in the sauce. Taste and adjust the seasoning.

7. Ladle the stew into the serving bowls.

8. Serve garnished with parsley.

Nutrition

Calories: 779

Fat: 41g

Carb: 31g

Protein: 67g

Provencal Braised Hake

Preparation Time: 10 minutes

Cooking Time: 20 minutes

Servings: 2

Ingredients

- Extra-virgin olive oil – 2 tbsp. plus extra for serving

- Onion – 1, halved and sliced thin

- Fennel bulb – 1, stalks discarded, bulb halved, cored and sliced thin
-
  Salt and black pepper
- Garlic clove – 4, minced

- Minced fresh thyme – 1 tsp.

- Diced tomatoes – 1 (14.5 ounce) can, drained

- Dry white wine – ½ cup

- Skinless hake fillets – 4 (4 to 6 ounce) 1 to 1 ½ inches thick

- Minced fresh parsley – 2 Tbsp.

Directions

1. Heat the oil in a skillet over medium heat. Add fennel, onion, and ½ tsp. salt and cook for 5 minutes. Stir in thyme and garlic and cook for 30 seconds.

2. Stir in the wine and tomatoes and then bring to a simmer.
3. Pat the hake dry with paper towels and season with salt and pepper. Place the hake into the skillet (skin side down). Spoon some sauce over the top and bring to a simmer.
4. Lower the heat to medium-low, cover, and cook for 10 to 12 minutes, or until the hake flakes apart when prodded with a knife.
5. Serve the hake into individual bowls. Stir parsley into the sauce and season with salt and pepper to taste. Spoon the sauce over the hake and drizzle with extra oil.
6. Serve.

Nutrition

Calories: 292

Fat: 11.1g

Carb: 11g

Protein: 33g

Pan-Roasted Sea Bass

Preparation Time: 5 minutes

Cooking Time: 10 minutes

Servings: 2

Ingredients

- Skinless sea bass fillets – 4 (4 to 6 ounces) 1 to 1 ½ inches thick

- Salt and pepper

- Sugar – ½ tsp.

- Extra-virgin olive oil – 1 tbsp.

- Lemon wedges

Directions

1. Place the oven rack in the middle and preheat the oven to 425F. Pat the sea bass dry with paper towels and season with salt and pepper. On one side of each fillet, sprinkle the sugar evenly.
2. In a skillet, heat the oil over medium-high. Place the sea bass sugared side down in the skillet and cook for 2 minutes, or until browned.
3. Then flip and transfer the skillet to the oven and roast for 7 to 10 minutes, or until the fish registers 140F.

4. Serve with lemon wedges.

Nutrition

Calories: 225

Fat: 4.3g

Carb: 1g

Protein: 45.5g

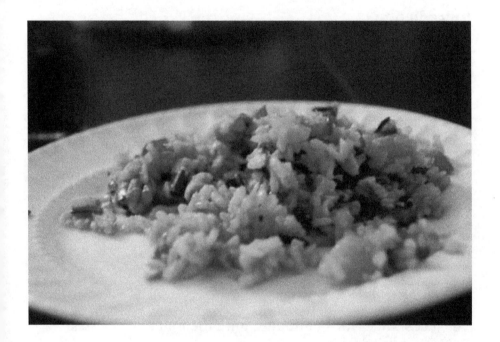

Delicious Quinoa & Dried

Preparation Time: 10 minutes

Cooking Time: 17 minutes

Servings: 2

Ingredients:

- 3 c. water
- ¼ c. cashew nut
- 8 dried apricots
- 4 dried figs
- 1 tsp. cinnamon

Directions:

1. In a pot, mix water and quinoa and
2. Let simmer for 15 minutes, until the water evaporates.
3. Chop dried fruit.
4. When quinoa is cooked, stir in all other ingredients.
5. Serve cold. Add milk, if desired.

Nutrition:

44g Carbs,

7g Fat,

13g Protein,

285 Calories 65

CPSIA information can be obtained
at www.ICGtesting.com
Printed in the USA
BVHW091455190521
607631BV00001B/218